I0436636

LIVER DETOX THERAPY

Treatment For Detoxification And Liver Health

Show Your Liver Some Love With Therapeutic Approaches That Enhance Detoxification And Support Liver Health

JAMES JOSEPH

CHAPTER ONE

Introduction

The human body is a complex and finely organized system, with numerous organs working together to ensure general health. Among these key organs, the liver stands out as a functioning powerhouse that plays an important role in overall health. Understanding the importance of liver health is critical for anybody hoping to improve their overall health and lifespan.

Understanding The Structure And Function Of The Liver

The liver is a big, reddish-brown organ found in the upper right side of the abdomen, under the ribcage. As the body's biggest internal organ, the liver is an unsung hero, providing a wide range of activities that contribute to general health. It is structurally split into two major lobes, which are further subdivided into smaller lobes called lobules.

The liver has several roles, including metabolic control, bile generation, and detoxification. Its involvement in metabolism includes controlling blood glucose levels, digesting nutrients taken from the digestive system, and storing important vitamins and minerals. Furthermore, the liver actively contributes to the creation of proteins required for blood coagulation and immunological function.

The Liver's Function In Detoxification

Detoxification is a basic function of the liver that includes the elimination of toxic chemicals from the body. The liver does this in two stages: phase I and phase II detoxification. Toxins are broken down into intermediate compounds by enzymes in phase I, and these intermediates are conjugated in Phase II to make them water-soluble and excretable.

Furthermore, the liver filters and processes blood from the digestive system before it circulates throughout the body. This guarantees that any potentially dangerous compounds absorbed by the intestines are neutralized or removed before they reach the other organs.

Liver Dysfunction Signs And Symptoms: Recognizing Warning Signs

Liver disease may present in a variety of ways, and identifying early warning symptoms is critical for appropriate management and preventing future consequences. Fatigue, unexplained weight loss, and changes in skin color, such as yellowing or darkening, are frequent signs of liver disease. Additionally, prolonged stomach discomfort and swelling, which are often accompanied by nausea and vomiting, may indicate underlying liver issues.

Changes in bowel habits, notably light-colored stools and black urine may potentially be signs of liver failure. It is important to pay attention to these symptoms, particularly if they continue for a long length of time, since they may indicate an underlying problem that needs medical intervention.

CHAPTER TWO
Common Health Concerns Associated With Liver Dysfunction

Liver dysfunction may come from a variety of circumstances, including viral infections and lifestyle decisions. Hepatitis, a common viral infection that causes inflammation of the liver, may result in acute or chronic liver disease. Alcohol-related liver damage is another common problem, generally caused by excessive and extended alcohol usage.

Non-alcoholic fatty liver disease (NAFLD) is becoming more common due to sedentary lifestyles and poor dietary choices. This disorder causes fat to accumulate in the liver, which may lead to inflammation and scarring. Cirrhosis, a severe and permanent scarring of the liver tissue, may arise from long-term liver malfunction, independent of the underlying cause.

Liver cancer, although less prevalent than other liver disorders, is a danger to overall health. It may develop as a primary cancer in the liver or as a secondary cancer that spreads to other regions of the body.

To summarize, knowing the significance of liver health is critical for general well-being. The liver's diverse involvement in metabolism, detoxification, and vital activities makes it an important part of the body's complex symphony of operations. Recognizing the signs and symptoms of liver dysfunction is critical for timely intervention and limiting the spread of liver-related health problems.

Regular medical check-ups, a healthy lifestyle, and careful use of chemicals that might harm liver health are all necessary components of keeping a robust and functional liver. Individuals may enhance longevity and live better lives by recognizing the liver's critical role in our health and making proactive efforts to support its well-being.

Diagnostic Tools For Liver Health.

Maintaining liver health is critical for general well-being, given the liver's important function in filtering pollutants, digesting nutrients, and facilitating digestion. Timely and precise tests are critical for monitoring liver function and identifying possible problems. Various diagnostic methods play an important role in monitoring liver health, giving essential information for preventative and treatment interventions.

Blood Tests And Liver Function

Blood tests that focus on liver function are one of the most common ways to assess liver health. Liver function tests, such as ALT, AST, and ALP, are routinely used to measure enzyme levels that indicate liver health. Elevated levels of these enzymes may indicate liver injury or inflammation, requiring additional examination.

Furthermore, evaluating bilirubin levels in the blood helps to assess the liver's capacity to process and eliminate waste products. High bilirubin levels may indicate problems with bile flow or metabolism, giving useful information for diagnosis and therapy planning.

Imaging Methods For Liver Assessment

Beyond blood testing, new imaging tools are critical for gaining a thorough knowledge of liver function. Non-invasive imaging techniques, such as ultrasound, computed tomography (CT) scans, and magnetic resonance imaging (MRI), enable healthcare practitioners to see the liver's structure, diagnose anomalies, and measure overall organ health.

Ultrasound is especially useful in identifying liver cirrhosis, malignancies, and irregular blood flow. CT scans provide comprehensive cross-sectional pictures, which help in the detection of liver tumors or abnormalities in surrounding tissues. MRI, with its greater soft tissue contrast, is useful for identifying liver lesions and determining the severity of liver disease.

These imaging tools not only help with diagnosis but also allow healthcare practitioners to track the evolution of liver disorders and assess the efficacy of therapy treatments.

CHAPTER THREE

Holistic Approaches To Liver Health

While diagnostic technologies are important for detecting liver problems, a comprehensive approach to liver health includes preventative treatments and lifestyle choices that may improve overall liver function.

Nutrition for Liver Support

Proper diet is essential for maintaining liver health. A well-balanced diet including a range of nutrients is critical for sustaining the liver's metabolic activities and fostering overall health. Antioxidant-rich diets, such as fruits and vegetables, assist to neutralize free radicals, which may cause liver damage.

Specific nutrients, such as vitamin E, C, and selenium, are essential for liver function. Nuts, seeds, citrus fruits, and leafy greens may all help to promote a nutrient-dense, liver-friendly diet.

Furthermore, avoiding processed foods, saturated fats, and excessive sweets is critical since they may overload the liver and lead to the development of non-alcoholic fatty liver disease (NAFLD). Individuals may actively contribute to liver health by eating mindfully and in moderation.

The Effect of Hydration on Liver Function

Adequate hydration is sometimes overlooked, although it plays an important role in sustaining liver function. Water is required for several body activities, including the removal of pollutants via urine and the maintenance of blood volume. Dehydration may cause concentrated bile, which may contribute to the production of gallstones and impair liver function.

A steady and adequate consumption of water throughout the day increases overall hydration, facilitates digestion, and supports the liver's natural detoxifying functions. This basic but important part of holistic liver care emphasizes the interdependence of lifestyle variables and organ function.

Detoxification Therapies

Detoxification treatments seek to improve the body's natural systems for removing toxins, with a particular emphasis on liver support. These treatments include lifestyle adjustments, dietary changes, and specific interventions aimed at improving liver function.

Regular exercise, for example, increases blood flow and enhances the effective digestion of nutrients and waste removal. Sweating during exercise promotes the outflow of toxins via the skin, providing an extra route for detoxification.

Sauna sessions have also become popular as a cleansing technique. The heat-induced sweating during sauna usage aids in the removal of toxins and may improve overall liver function. However, such treatments should be approached with prudence, taking into account specific health issues and talking with healthcare specialists before adopting them into a wellness regimen.

Furthermore, some dietary regimens, such as intermittent fasting or a liver cleanse diet, are thought to aid in detoxification. However, empirical data on the effectiveness and safety of these methods is mixed, highlighting the significance of tailored procedures under expert supervision.

Finally, diagnostic tools for liver health, such as blood testing and imaging procedures, give vital insights into the liver's condition and help guide medical actions. However, a comprehensive approach to liver health, including diet, hydration, and detoxification therapy, is essential for maintaining good liver function and avoiding possible problems. By combining diagnostic precision with proactive lifestyle choices, people may actively contribute to the well-being of this crucial organ and promote long-term health.

Herbal Treatments For Liver Detox

The liver is a critical organ in the human body that plays an important role in detoxification and general health. Poor dietary choices, exposure to environmental pollutants, and sedentary lifestyles may all put a burden on the liver's functioning. Herbal medicines have long been acknowledged for their ability to promote liver function and help in detoxification.

One of the most effective methods to boost liver health via herbal means is to include particular herbs into one's daily regimen. Milk thistle, a well-known plant, is often praised for its capacity to preserve and regenerate the liver. Silymarin, the main ingredient in milk thistle, has antioxidant and anti-inflammatory effects that may help regenerate liver cells and protect against free radical damage.

Turmeric, another potent plant, includes curcumin, which has been widely researched for its anti-inflammatory and antioxidant properties. According to research, turmeric may assist in lowering liver inflammation and preventing liver disease. Including turmeric in one's diet or taking it as a supplement may be a natural method to promote liver function.

Dandelion root is also known for its ability to stimulate liver cleansing. It is thought to promote bile production, which helps with fat digestion and breakdown. Dandelion root also contains diuretic qualities, which may help to eliminate toxins from the liver and kidneys.

Artichoke leaf extract, another herbal medicine, has been examined for its liver-protective properties. It is supposed to stimulate bile flow, which aids in the liver's natural detoxifying operations. Regular use of artichoke leaf extract may improve liver function.

CHAPTER FOUR

The Benefits Of Juicing For Liver Health

Juicing is becoming more popular as a technique of giving a concentrated dosage of nutrients to the body, and it may be especially good for liver function. Freshly squeezed juices from fruits and vegetables may give the liver with necessary vitamins, minerals, and antioxidants to aid in detoxification.

Beet juice, for example, contains betalains and antioxidants that may help decrease inflammation and promote liver detoxification. Nitrates in beets are turned into nitric oxide, which improves blood flow and oxygen supply to the liver.

Carrot juice is another wonderful choice since it contains beta-carotene and other antioxidants that enhance liver function. The body converts beta-carotene into vitamin A, which helps the liver operate.

Green leafy vegetables, such as kale and spinach, maybe juiced to receive chlorophyll, a chemical that may help with liver detoxification by neutralizing toxins. Green juices also include a lot of vitamins and minerals, which might help your liver stay healthy.

While juicing may be a beneficial supplement to a liver-friendly diet, it is critical to balance it with whole foods and eat a diversified and well-rounded diet for optimal nutritional results.

Fasting Protocols And Their Effect On The Liver

Intermittent fasting and other fasting regimes have received attention due to their potential advantages, which include enhanced metabolic health and weight control. Interestingly, fasting may have a favorable impact on liver health and function.

During fasting, the body switches from utilizing glucose as its major energy source to burning stored fat. This metabolic flip may alleviate the stress on the liver, which is in charge of digesting and storing extra glucose as glycogen before turning it back into glucose when required.

Intermittent fasting, which involves alternating periods of eating and fasting, may improve the liver's capacity to metabolize lipids and manage blood sugar levels. This process, known as autophagy, involves the body breaking down and eliminating damaged cells, which may aid liver detoxification.

Extended fasting, such as water or juice fasting, may produce more significant liver benefits. During prolonged fasting, the body enters a condition of ketosis, which causes the breakdown of fat cells in the liver. This technique may help reduce liver fat and enhance liver function.

However, fasting should be approached with care and under supervision, particularly for those who have pre-existing health concerns. It is recommended that you consult with a healthcare practitioner before starting any fasting program.

Lifestyle Changes For Liver Wellness

Maintaining a healthy lifestyle is essential for liver fitness. Lifestyle decisions such as regular exercise, stress management, and avoiding dangerous drugs all play important roles in liver health.

Exercise's Role in Liver Health

Regular physical exercise provides several health advantages, including improved liver function. Exercise promotes a healthy weight and lowers the risk of nonalcoholic fatty liver disease (NAFLD).

Aerobic activity, such as brisk walking, jogging, or cycling, may boost blood circulation and increase oxygen supply to the liver. This increased blood flow aids the liver's cleansing and general function.

Resistance or strength exercise is also good for liver health. Increasing muscle mass may increase insulin sensitivity, lowering the risk of metabolic disorders that can lead to liver problems.

Stress Management For Healthy Liver

Chronic stress has a deleterious influence on many facets of health, including liver function. When the body is stressed, it produces chemicals such as cortisol, which, if chronically increased, may cause inflammation and liver damage.

Integrating stress management tactics into your daily routine might be critical for keeping a healthy liver. Mindfulness meditation, deep breathing exercises, and yoga are all effective ways to decrease stress and improve general well-being.

Getting enough sleep is another crucial part of stress management. Quality sleep enables the body to repair and rejuvenate, which promotes healthy liver function. Establishing a regular sleep schedule and providing a pleasant nighttime atmosphere may help to improve sleep quality.

Medical Interventions For Liver Support

In certain circumstances, medicinal measures may be required to maintain liver health. These treatments include drugs for treating liver problems and surgical techniques to treat particular liver illnesses.

Medications And Liver Health

Certain drugs may affect liver function, either favorably or adversely. Individuals must be aware of the possible effects of drugs on the liver and consult with healthcare specialists as needed.

For example, some drugs, such as those used to treat diabetes or excessive cholesterol, may have an impact on liver function. Regular monitoring and discussion with healthcare experts may assist ensure that drugs are taken properly, particularly given their possible influence on the liver.

In situations of liver illnesses or problems, healthcare providers may prescribe drugs that treat the underlying concerns. Antiviral medicines for hepatitis infections and immunosuppressants for autoimmune liver illnesses are two examples of such therapies.

CHAPTER FIVE

Surgical Intervention And Liver Disorders

Surgical treatments may be considered in cases when liver problems need more severe therapy. Liver transplantation is a common option for those with end-stage liver disease or liver failure.

During a liver transplant, a damaged liver is replaced with a healthy donor liver. This operation may be life-saving for those with serious liver diseases and provides a chance for a new and better life.

Other surgical operations may involve tumor removal or the treatment of particular structural abnormalities in the liver. These therapies are intended to ease symptoms, prevent additional damage, and enhance overall liver function.

To summarize, sustaining liver health requires a complex strategy that includes herbal medicines, dietary choices, lifestyle changes, and, if required, medical procedures. By implementing these tactics into their everyday lives, people may help their liver's natural detoxification processes and improve their overall health. It is important to contact healthcare specialists for specific advice and direction, particularly when contemplating major lifestyle changes or medicinal procedures for liver health.

Alternative Treatments For Liver Love

The liver is a critical organ that performs detoxification, metabolism, and a variety of other necessary tasks in the human body. While medical treatments are essential for treating liver disorders, alternative therapies may supplement standard procedures and improve overall liver health. Acupuncture, based on

Traditional Chinese Medicine, and Ayurvedic liver cleaning are two famous alternative treatments.

According to TCM, the liver is responsible for the smooth flow of qi throughout the body. Acupuncture seeks to balance this energy flow and promotes healthy liver function.

According to studies, acupuncture may offer advantages for liver health. According to research, acupuncture may help decrease inflammation, increase blood circulation, and boost liver function indicators. Furthermore, acupuncture treatments are often accompanied by lifestyle suggestions, such as dietary adjustments and stress management techniques, which contribute to overall liver health.

Ayurvedic Approaches to Liver Cleansing: Ayurveda, a historic Indian medical philosophy, promotes overall well-being and equilibrium. Ayurvedic liver health methods entail cleaning and detoxifying the liver to keep it functioning optimally. Ayurvedic liver treatment relies heavily on herbal therapies, dietary adjustments, and lifestyle recommendations.

Turmeric, a frequently used spice in Ayurveda, includes curcumin, which has anti-inflammatory and antioxidant effects. Turmeric may improve liver function by lowering inflammation and guarding against oxidative damage. Ayurvedic practitioners also propose certain dietary recommendations, such as eating bitter and astringent foods, which are thought to help with liver cleansing.

Preventing Liver Damage

Preventing liver disease is critical to sustaining overall health. Understanding the effects of alcohol, as well as implementing hepatitis prevention and immunization methods, are two critical components of liver damage prevention.

Alcohol and Liver Health: Excessive alcohol intake is a major cause of liver damage and illness, including alcoholic liver disease and cirrhosis. The liver metabolizes alcohol, and persistent alcohol misuse may cause inflammation, fatty liver, and irreparable damage. Understanding the effects of alcohol on liver health is critical for avoiding alcohol-related liver damage.

It is important to educate people about the benefits of moderate alcohol intake as well as the hazards of excessive drinking. Public health campaigns and awareness initiatives play an important role in encouraging appropriate alcohol consumption, lowering liver load, and minimizing long-term harm.

Hepatitis Prevention and Vaccination: Viral hepatitis, especially hepatitis B and C, is a major hazard to liver health. Preventing hepatitis infections is critical to preventing liver damage and its consequences. Vaccination against hepatitis B is an important preventative strategy, particularly in areas where the infection is widespread.

Routine vaccination, particularly for at-risk groups such as healthcare professionals, those with many sexual partners, and those who engage in high-risk behaviors, may considerably lower the prevalence of hepatitis B. Additionally, practicing safe sex, avoiding sharing needles, and taking measures against bloodborne illnesses all help to prevent hepatitis.

CHAPTER SIX

Maintaining Liver Health In Specific Populations.

The liver's health varies by age group, hence specialized treatments are required for various populations such as children and the elderly.

Pediatric Liver Health: Children may be impacted by a variety of liver issues, including congenital and metabolic illnesses. Promoting a balanced diet, frequent exercise, and appropriate vaccines are all important ways to maintain juvenile liver health. Early identification and intervention are critical in the efficient management and treatment of liver problems.

Educating parents and caregivers on the significance of a liver-friendly lifestyle for their children, including diet and immunization, is critical for ensuring optimum liver health from a young age.

Senior Liver Wellness: As people become older, their livers alter, making them more susceptible to certain liver disorders. Seniors may be at risk for non-alcoholic fatty liver disease (NAFLD) and age-related liver disorders. Healthy lifestyle choices such as a well-balanced diet, frequent exercise, and moderate alcohol use help to preserve senior liver health.

Routine health screenings for seniors should include liver function testing to enable for early diagnosis of possible problems. Furthermore, healthcare experts may advise elders on drugs and supplements that may affect liver function, allowing them to make more educated decisions about their overall well-being.

Real-Life Success Stories

Individuals battling liver health difficulties might be inspired and encouraged by real-life success stories. Personal paths to liver health often include a mix of medical treatments, alternative therapies, and lifestyle adjustments.

Personal Journeys to Liver Health: These tales include people who have overcome liver health difficulties, demonstrating the power of perseverance and a dedication to a liver-friendly lifestyle. Success stories may involve acupuncture, Ayurvedic treatments, and following medical advice.

Individuals dealing with liver health difficulties might be encouraged and motivated to make good changes in their lives by sharing these stories. Real-life success stories support the idea that taking a complete approach to liver health has beneficial consequences.

Conclusion

Adopting a liver-friendly lifestyle is essential for general health, and alternative therapies may supplement traditional medical treatments. Acupuncture and Ayurvedic approaches to liver health provide holistic viewpoints, stressing the significance of energy balance and natural cleansing.

Understanding the influence of alcohol on liver health is essential for preventing liver damage, as is adopting hepatitis prevention and immunization methods. Tailoring techniques for particular populations, such as children and the elderly, ensures that patients get complete treatment throughout all ages.

Real-life success stories are beacons of hope, demonstrating the transformational impact of leading a liver-friendly lifestyle. Individuals with liver health difficulties might find inspiration and motivation to improve their health by sharing their stories. Finally, a well-balanced strategy that incorporates medical treatment, alternative therapies, and a dedication to a liver-friendly lifestyle improves the liver's general health and vitality.

www.ingramcontent.com/pod-product-compliance
Lightning Source LLC
Chambersburg PA
CBHW071218290526
45796CB00008B/282